I0435214

KEEP YOUR KIDS FIT

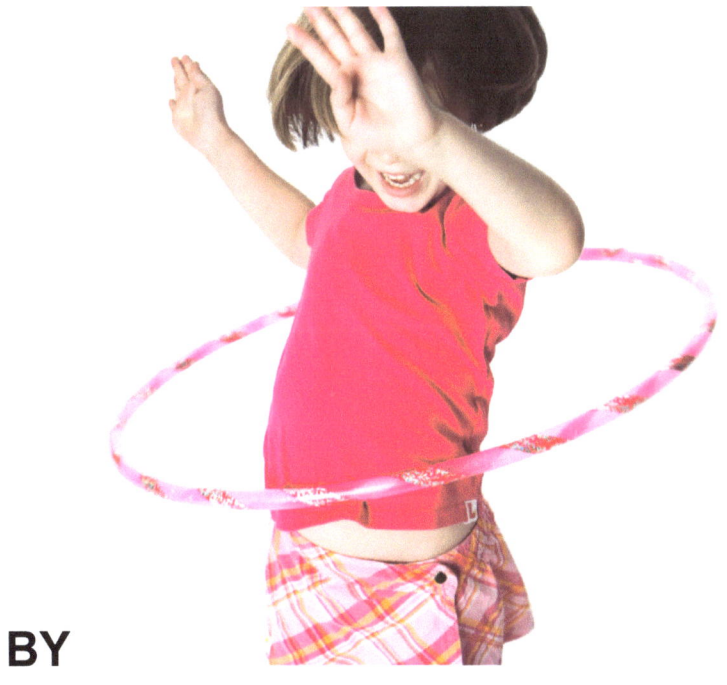

BY

Dr. Carleen Varga, MSN

Educating your children on understanding food intake is important.
The target age starts between 5 years-12 years.
Nutrition education is important and can alleviate some of the poor health statistics.

The following contents are as follows:

Ojectives

Content

Learning Objectives

Life Skills

Facts

Risks and Diseases

Food Choices

Go, Slow, Stop Foods

Title of Activity: Life Skills: Keep your Kids Fit For Life – Diet

Total Number of Contact Hours: One

Intended Level of Learner: Basic

Purpose/Goal: To understand the health risks of childhood obesity, recognize unhealthy eating behaviors and learn healthy eating choices for life.

Objectives	Content (Topics)	Teaching/Learning Resources
List why childhood overweight (obesity) is a problem.	What contributes to Obesity --Statistics - Risks and diseases -- Ideal body weight	Written material online Reference material Post test
Describe healthy eating	What kind of eating makes kids overweight? Healthy eating guidelines	Written material online Activity Reference material Post test
List healthy eating choices for meals, snacks, and eating out	Tips from parents	Written material online Reference material Post test

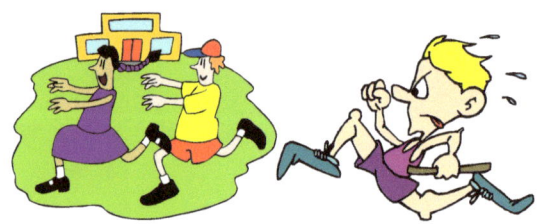

Life Skills: Keep Kids Fit For Life – Diet

By
Dr.Carleen Varga, RN, MSN, Nutritionist,
Previous Owner of Fitwize 4 Kids

Introduction: Children in the United States are at risk of serious health problems due to their weight. Parents need to help children make healthy choices in what they eat.

Topic 1: Childhood Obesity – a growing problem

Topic Description: Being overweight is called "obesity". Being overweight is not healthy. People who are overweight are at risk for certain diseases. It is important that both children and parents learn how to make healthy eating choices.

Facts

Children in the U.S. are growing more and more overweight. 17% of all school aged children weigh too much, according to a study by the Centers for Disease Control (CDC). Thirty years ago, only 4% of children were overweight. Notice in the chart how the problem has grown over the years.

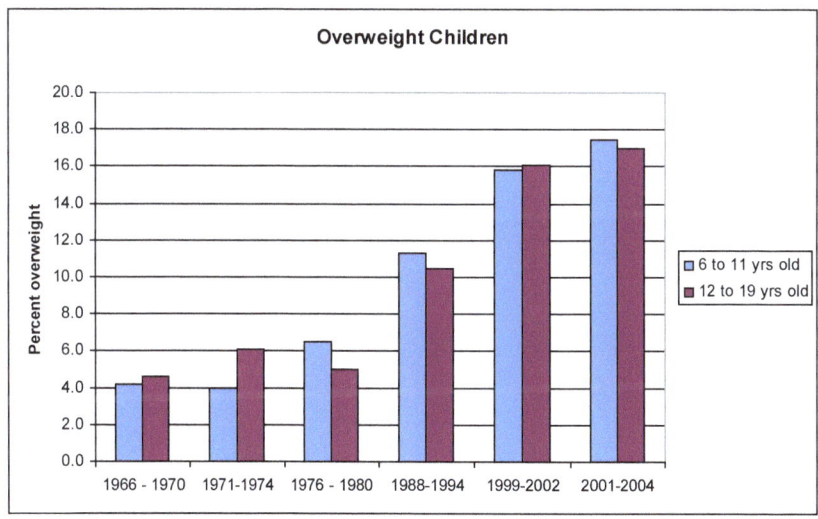

Risks and Diseases

Risk factors for disease are very high in children who are overweight. Overweight children are at higher risk of:

- Diabetes
- High blood pressure
- Asthma and other breathing problems
- Sleep disorders
- Liver disease
- Early puberty (girls starting their periods early)
- Eating disorders
- Skin infections

Overweight teenagers have a 70% chance of becoming overweight adults. That jumps to 80% if one or both parents are overweight. In adults, being overweight can also lead to a greater risk of some forms of cancer, stroke, and other diseases.

The overweight child not only has health risks, but is more likely to be depressed and have poor self-esteem. Being overweight can cause:

- **Low self-esteem and bullying.** Children often tease or bully children who are overweight
- **Behavior and learning problems.** Overweight children tend to have more anxiety and poorer social skills than normal-weight children have. This may lead to acting badly at school or it may cause the child to stay away from other children and have few friends. Stress and anxiety also make it hard for the child to learn, leading to poor grades.
- **Depression.** Social isolation and low self-esteem can cause children to lose hope that their lives will improve. This can lead to depression. A depressed child may lose interest in normal activities, sleep more than usual or cry a lot. Depression is as serious in children as in adults.

Causes of Childhood Overweight

The diseases caused by being overweight don't happen quickly. These diseases gradually build up over time. You might not see these things happening right away, so there is not an instant connection to unhealthy eating. But over time, problems will set in. For example, what if you did not change the oil in your car? At first, the car would run as usual. As time went on, you would notice problems, and eventually the car would stop running and need to go to the shop for repairs.

Here are the main reasons that children are overweight:

- Poor eating habits
- Lack of exercise

It's as simple as that: too much to eat and too little exercise. So, it's up to you to work with your child to keep him at a healthy body weight. We have some easy tips for you to start using today, as well as handouts to print and tape to the refrigerator at home. Start now! Your child will thank you later as a healthy young woman or young man.

How much should your child weigh?

The ideal body weight for children is not a "one size fits all" description. For children 2 years old to 19 years old, the best way to check for ideal weight is with the BMI – Body Mass Index. BMI ranges for children and teens take into account normal differences in body fat between boys and girls and differences in body fat as they grow. It's not as easy as a chart that lists height and ideal weight, because healthy weight ranges change every month as children grow.

Here's an activity for you to try right away. Check your child's BMI at the Center for Disease Control's BMI Calculator. You will need to type in your child's height, birthday, and weight. Try it now:

http://apps.nccd.cdc.gov/dnpabmi/Calculator.aspx

Some times the way a child is raised also affects her weight. Some groups of people have traditions of foods that are tasty but are high in fat or high in calories. How much money parents have to spend on food can also affect the food choices that parents make. Look at the chart below and see if you notice groups of children that are more likely to be overweight than some other children.

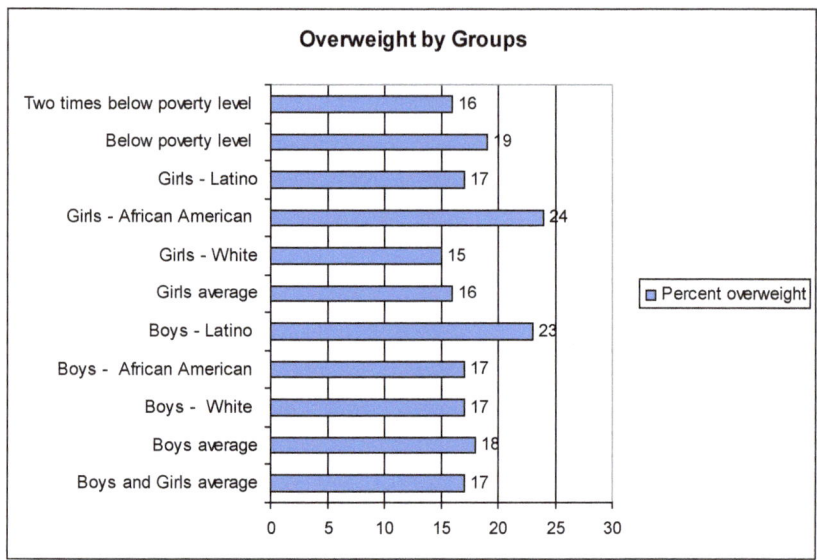

Chart data from CDC http://www.cdc.gov/nchs/data/hus/hus06.pdf#074

Activity: who is more at risk for overweight?

In the chart you just looked at, which group is more likely to be overweight?

- Latino Girls
- **Latino Boys**
- **African American Girls**
- African American Boys

Summary

Being overweight can have serious problems for your child, including disease and depression. Poor eating and lack of exercise are the main reasons children are overweight.

Topic 2: Healthy Eating

Topic Description: To make healthy eating choices, you and your child need to know what makes up healthy eating.   In this section we will compare foods that are good, almost good, and bad choices for healthy eating, as well as other ideas to keep a healthy weight for your child.

Non-healthy choices

Check the list below to see if your child is making one or more of these non-healthy choices:

- Eating high fat food
- Eating too much sugar
- Eating fewer fresh vegetables, fruits, and whole-grain foods
- Eating too much – large plates at meals and snacks
- Watching TV or playing video games for too long
- Not exercising at least 30 minutes a day
- Not getting enough information on healthy eating to make good choices

In this course, we will give you some easy to use ideas for helping your child make healthy choices. Each of these ideas is explained with examples. At the end of the course, there are Internet sites with more tips for you and your child.

Healthy choices:
1. **Eat fruits, vegetables, and whole grains every day**
2. **Always eat breakfast**
3. **Watch out for WHOA FOODS**
4. **Limit screen or TV time to 2 hours per day**
5. **Be active every day**
6. **Drink lots of water**
7. **Pay attention**

1. **Eat fruits, vegetables, and whole grains every day.**
Children should eat fruit and vegetables every day. As parents, we need to offer fruit and vegetables to our children. Whole grains are great choices to eat, as they provide bulk and help children to eat less. It's fairly easy to tell a fresh fruit or vegetable, but what is a whole grain?

What to look for on the food label to find whole grains:

Choose foods that name one of the following whole-grain ingredients *first* on the label's ingredient list:

"brown rice"   "whole oats"
"bulgur"   "whole rye"
"graham flour"   "whole wheat"
"oatmeal"   "wild rice"
"whole-grain corn"

- Foods labeled with the words "multi-grain," "stone-ground," "100% wheat," "cracked wheat," "seven-grain," or "bran" are usually *not* whole-grain.
- Brown color doesn't mean it is whole grain. Bread can be brown because of molasses or other added ingredients. Read the food label to see if it is a whole grain.
- Use the food label and choose products with a higher amount of **fiber.** Fiber is a good clue to the amount of whole grain in the product.

Tips to help you eat whole grains

- Try brown rice, whole wheat pasta or whole wheat macaroni
- Use barley in soup or stews
- Use whole-grain bread or oats in meatloaf instead of white bread
- Try oats or a crushed, unsweetened whole grain cereal as breading for baked chicken, fish, veal cutlets, or eggplant parmesan
- Snack on ready-to-eat, whole grain cereals such as toasted oat cereal.
- Try a whole-grain snack chip, such as baked tortilla chips.
- Popcorn, a whole grain, can be a healthy snack with little or no added salt and butter
- Let children choose and help fix a whole grain side dish
- Teach older children to read the food label on cereals or snack food packages and choose those with whole grains at the top of the list

2. **Always Eat Breakfast**

This is the easiest meal to skip. Make a rule in your home that everyone eats breakfast every day. Choose whole grain cereal with milk, oatmeal, eggs, cottage cheese or yogurt for a good start that includes protein and whole grains. Children can pay attention better in school with a healthy breakfast to fuel their brains.

Are you too busy in the morning to cook breakfast? Make up breakfast burritos the night before and wrap them up in the refrigerator for a quick breakfast with fruit and milk the next morning. Don't skip breakfast!

3. Watch out for WHOA FOODS

Learn how to choose healthy foods for your kids: the Go, Slow, and Whoa foods.

Here's an easy way to teach your child how to choose foods that are good for him.

GO foods: go through a green light (eat all of these you would like)
SLOW foods: slow down on the yellow light (don't eat as much of these)
WHOA foods: stop on the red light (eat these foods only once in a while)

Here is a chart for you to print and post at home with Go, Slow, and Whoa choices. Put the chart on your refrigerator and take a look at this from time to time. Bring it with you to the grocery store and ask your child to help you choose snacks for the next week.

Food Group	GO	SLOW	WHOA
Fruit	**Fresh is best, unpeeled** Frozen - no sugar Canned fruit in its own juice Dried fruit no sugar added	Fruit juice Dried fruit, sugar added	Canned fruit in heavy syrup
Vegetables	**Fresh is best, unpeeled** Frozen - no sauce	Sauces on vegetables	Fried
Bread, grains	Whole grain bread Cereal – look for "made with whole grains" Corn tortilla Brown rice Whole grain pasta	White bread Biscuits, rolls Pancakes Granola Taco shells White rice Regular pasta	Croissants Doughnuts Muffins Cookies Sweetened cereal
Dairy	Fat free yogurt Fat free cottage cheese Fat free sour cream	Ice milk or slow churned, less fat ice cream Frozen yogurt	Whole milk cheese Ice cream
Meat	Lean beef Lean pork Tuna in water Chicken – white meat, no skin Turkey – white meat, no skin	Ham Canadian Bacon Turkey dark meat, skin Chicken dark meat, skin Tuna in oil	Bacon Ribs Fried meat of any kind Hot Dogs Lunch Meats Pepperoni Sausage
Sweets, Snacks	Ice Milk Frozen fruit bars Fig bars, ginger snaps Baked potato chips Low fat popcorn Pretzels	Angel food cake Ice cream low fat slow churned	Cake Pie Cheesecake Potato Chips Candy Buttered popcorn
Drinks	Water Unsweetened lemonade Fat free or 1% milk	100% Fruit Juice 2% milk Sports drink Diet Soda	Regular soda Whole milk Sweetened lemonade Fruit drink (not juice)

11

Smart choices – GO foods - are the foods with the lowest amounts of fat or added sugar. For example, choose fat-free (skim) milk instead of whole milk and unsweetened rather than sweetened applesauce. Also, look at how the food was cooked. Choose skinless baked chicken instead of fried chicken. Choose the broiled fish sandwich instead of the fried fish sandwich.   And remember that fresh is best. Choose an apple before apple sauce. It's easy!

ACTIVITY:

Make the healthy choice: <pictures would be great for this activity>

baked yam	mashed potatoes
orange juice	**fresh orange**
cheese slices	chips with queso

Low fat and reduced fat – what does it mean?

Choosing lower-fat foods is a healthy way to eat, but buying lower-fat foods can be confusing. Here is what the labels mean:

One serving:

Fat-free	Less than half a gram of fat
Low fat	3 grams or less fat
Reduced or less fat	At least 25% less fat*
Light	One-third fewer calories and/or 50% less fat*

* Compared to a serving of the traditional food

As always, read the food label. Low fat does not always mean low calorie. To make the food low fat, sometimes sugar and other high-calorie foods are added. Also watch portion size. It's easy to eat twice as much "because it's low fat".

For those of you who tried low fat foods and found them tasteless, try again. Food companies have worked hard to make these foods tastier, creamier and more satisfying. Try different brands, as one company may make a better low fat sour cream, for example, than another company. Give low fat a try!

4. **Limit TV time to 2 hours per day.**

Hours of screen time is linked to weight gain, so limit TV time to no more than two hours a day. Always keep the television, video games and computer out of the bedroom. Put the TV, computer and videogame console where you can see them. This way you can keep track of not only how much, but what, your children are doing.

5. **Be Active Every Day**

Everyone should be active every day. This doesn't just mean exercise at a gym. It means playing, walking, running – anything that gets you moving. A great way to add activity to your life is to do things as a family. Walk the dog together, rake leaves, or wash windows – anything to keep moving. Being physically active is a key to living a longer, healthier, happier life. Physical activity can also help you achieve and maintain a healthy weight and lower risk for disease. The benefits of physical activity may include:
- Improves self-esteem
- Helps build bones, muscles, and joints
- Helps manage weight
- Lowers risk of heart disease, colon cancer, and type 2 diabetes
- Helps control blood pressure
- Reduces feelings of depression and anxiety

Physical activity and eating well work together for better health. Being active increases the amount of calories burned, which helps keep weight at a healthy level.

6. **Drink lots of water every day.**

Sodas have 150 calories **per can.** That's a lot of empty calories with no vitamins, minerals or anything else good for your body. Water is always a good choice. Milk is good, too, as is 100% fruit or vegetable juice. Watch out for sugar-added drinks. Sometimes a diet soda can be a sweet but low-calorie treat. However, it is an empty treat, with no vitamins or minerals. Offer your child milk, juice or water.

7. **Pay attention.**

A big part of learning to eat well is paying attention not only to what you eat but also when you eat. It's easy to eat hundreds of calories without even knowing it – and often without enjoying the food you are eating. How many times have you eaten a snack while watching TV, only to look at the empty snack bowl and not remember eating all of it? Teach your child about paying attention, especially:

- Eating while watching TV or playing videogames
- Eating while reading or studying
- Eating while in the car

TIPS: Teach your child to pay attention while eating by talking about how the food tastes, saying "this cottage cheese is creamy, isn't it?", or "the yogurt reminds me of ice cream".

Tell your child to chew slowly, at least 20 times for each bite of food, and to lay their fork down between bites. The feeling of being "full" takes time. Children who eat fast, eat more.

Choose different kinds of foods for each meal – crunchy, smooth, chewy, sweet, and salty. Example: pork chops (chewy, salty) with sweet potatoes (smooth, sweet) and salad (crunchy, lots of different flavors).

Paying attention also applies to you as a parent. Pay attention to what your child eats. Pay attention to what snacks are in the house. Pay attention to the menu for school lunches, and talk to your child about choices to make for lunch if she buys lunch at school. Last, but not least, pay attention to what you eat. Be a role model for your child. That's the best way to teach your child healthy choices.

Summary: Making good food choices and staying active can help your child stay healthy.

Topic 3: Healthy eating choices for meals, snacks, special occasions and eating out

Topic Description: This section will give you ideas for making healthy meals and snacks. This is not "dieting", just some changes in the way you eat now in order to maintain a healthy lifestyle.   Here are some ideas from other families that I have worked with that you can use. Many are tips from moms and dads who found healthy ways to help their children eat well.

Never Empty Veggie Platter

My kids are ravenous when they come home from school. If I am not careful they eat too many snacks and don't want any dinner. One of our favorite healthy snacks is the Never Empty Veggie Platter. I cut up carrots, celery, sugar snap peas, broccoli, lightly steamed green beans and include a dip made from cottage cheese and Ranch salad dressing whirred up in the blender. They eat that very willingly.

Ants on a Hill

We have a family snack called Ants on a Hill. Cut up pieces of celery and let your kids spread peanut butter on the celery and then add raisins. These are very nutritious and full of fiber. Another treat we like is plain yogurt with cut up pieces of fruit to mix in. You even can sprinkle some granola on top to get at least 3 food groups.

Proteins and Carbs

I feed five children after school. Kid favorites are cheese and crackers, veggies with dip, granola bars, animal crackers or pretzels (buy the giant 3 pound bag at the warehouse to save money), and graham crackers with peanut butter. Of course, my group does like fruit, so I give them bananas, melon etc. I try to avoid concentrated sweets like cookies or candy. The theme for us seems to mix some protein and carbs to last. Snacks get washed down with milk if there is not a lot of protein in the snack.

Start With Tortillas

Great healthy snacks start with inexpensive tortillas. My kids like a little grated cheese melted on a tortilla. I fold it and cut it in wedges. They dip it in salsa. If your kids don't like salsa, it is good plain. We have also used leftovers like tuna or egg salad, sloppy joe filling, peanut butter and jelly, or chili to fill the tortillas. I think the reason they like them so much is the small triangle shapes. It is very easy to heat any of these when they are needed.

Dried Fruit and Nuts

A very delicious and healthy snack is nuts (unsalted) mixed with raisins, chopped dates or any favorite dried fruit. I usually have raisins, dates, walnuts, and almonds. This is a good snack for the entire family. I also make hot/spicy and a pumpkin pie spice version by adding spices and stirring.

Mini-Pizzas

We usually don't eat dinner until late so a rather hardy snack is nice for my kids when they come home from school hungry. I like to take some spare time on a weekend to make up a big batch of mini pizzas and freeze them individually. The ingredients are very simple:

a tube of refrigerator biscuits
canned pizza sauce
shredded cheese

You can add any other toppings you want. I like to use thin slices of hot dogs. Inexpensive thin sliced ham or any lunchmeat also works well. Of course, pepperoni is a favorite. Just smash the biscuits flat, top them however you want, bake them until the cheese melts and they look done. This usually takes about 8 minutes, depending on how much topping you use. The items you buy for toppings really go a long way because it only takes a little for each biscuit.

These mini pizzas can be reheated in the microwave for a few seconds for a great after school snack. My husband works second shift so I even make him his own batch with hot peppers and mushrooms for his after work snack!

Kids' Choice

We take a six-cupcake pan and put a different treat in each cupcake spot. Some choices include: cheese cubes, vegetables, cereal, raisins or fruit, yogurt, pretzels, crackers, nuts, pieces of bagel etc. The kids like the fact that they have a wide array of things and can pick and choose. What isn't used is covered and the following day we add new selections. Sometimes I end up having to eat things that have been passed over for two days, but I find my kids eating more healthy options and being refueled after a long day without spoiling their appetite for dinner.

Kids' Kabobs

One snack my 3 girls like is mini fruit and cheese kabobs. Using toothpicks as skewers, thread on fruit and cheese of your choice. Mine like pineapple, strawberries and chunks of mozzarella. Or try grapes, cheddar and apples. The choices are endless and you can cater to each child's taste. I make a big batch and put them in the fridge. They never lasted long. If your children are very young watch the toothpicks!

Healthy Treats at Home - Snacks

- Rice cakes with peanut butter. Try mini-rice cakes for a kid-sized treat
- Whole wheat crackers with cheese and grapes
- Pretzels instead of potato chips
- Apple slices and cheese

- Fruit cut up or on skewers served with low fat yogurt dip
- Vegetable trays served with low fat ranch, hummus or cottage cheese.
- Yogurt parfait bar - use several flavors of low fat yogurt with add-ins such as granola, whole wheat cheerios, uncooked oatmeal, raisins, dried fruit or nuts
- Have half sandwiches ready made for snacks

Dinner Ideas

- Wrap it up -   tortillas can be wrapped with cream cheese, shredded carrots, cucumber slices, turkey or ham
- Quick Salad -- serve a large salad with cold chicken chunks and light ranch dressing
- Soup Samples - Serve tea cups of different kinds of soup, with a piece of fresh fruit or celery sticks and whole grain crackers.
- Taco night - Serve corn tortillas, blue chips, chicken, refried beans, lettuce, tomatoes, salsa, avocado and fat free sour cream
- Pasta Night - toss any cooked pasta (wheat or fortified is best) with chopped tomatoes, fresh shredded basil and cubes of mozzarella cheese, chopped black olives and toss with balsamic vinaigrette or any Italian dressing.
- Greek Platter- on a large platter, place hummus, sun dried tomatoes, olives, feta cheese, and canned tuna. If your kids like them, try anchovies on the platter, too.   Serve with a large Greek salad and pita bread.
- "To Go" Night - order sides of spaghetti or ravioli from your favorite restaurant, serve in ONE CUP PORTIONS with a salad and a side of fruit.

Healthy choices when eating out, special events, and holidays.

Eating out is a challenge, especially at a fast food restaurant. There are so many high fat choices but there are also some healthier choices you can make and still enjoy the food. Instead of French fries, have a baked potato or salad instead. Instead of a soft drink, substitute milk or water. Order a hamburger instead of a cheeseburger, and ask to have it your way, with no mayonnaise. Order a wrap if it's on the menu, for less bread. Order broiled, not fried. Order low fat salad dressing. And don't forget that you can ask for a menu with calories and fat listed – the "food label" of fast food. This can help you make better choices. Many fast food restaurants are now offering healthy side choices for children such as apple slices and low fat milk. This makes it easier for you and your child to make a good choice. Check online for calories in fast food. Most fast food websites have an online menu with food label information listed.

"If we could give every individual the right amount of nourishment and exercise, not too little and not too much, we would have found the safest way to health."
Hippocrates

Special events – parties, holidays, and family gatherings – can be a tough time to make healthy food choices. What do you do about all those goodies? Grandma's fried chicken, your sister's special cheesecake, and the bowls of potato chips and dip are all there for the eating. The good news is, you and your child can have a treat now and then. The trick is to take less of the high calorie food, and more of the salad and vegetables. And, of course, not to eat those special foods very often.

TIP: "It's the weekend".
Save desserts for the weekend. Don't serve them during the week. Make them a treat for a time when the family is together. During the week, desserts are a WHOA food, but on Saturday and Sunday, you can say "It's the weekend" and have a treat. Of course, your best choice is a lower-fat, lower-sugar dessert. Here are some ideas:

Angel food cake with fruit

Slice fresh fruit and sprinkle it with a little sugar. Let the fruit sit in the bowl for half an hour to draw out the fruit's natural sugar. It will make a lovely "sauce" with the fruit. Spoon over angel food cake slices. Heavenly!

Frozen grapes
Wash and dry seedless grapes. Dip them in a little sugar, and then spread them on a pan or plate, and place in the freezer for an hour. Fun and delicious.

Frozen Bananas
Cut bananas in half. Place a Popsicle stick in each half and freeze overnight. Dip in melted chocolate and chopped nuts and enjoy! (Some grocery stores sell frozen banana kits in the produce department)

Baked Apples
Core apples and fill with raisins and brown sugar. Bake at 350 for half an hour.

Final Tip: Watch the size – portion control

Here are some ways to cut the amount your child eats.

- Serve up the meal to your child with the right amount of food already on the plate. Leave the serving dishes in the kitchen, and use the leftovers for another meal rather than a second helping.
- Use a smaller plate. For kids, this can be fun. Buy cute plates at the dollar store, making sure they are smaller than your usual dinner plates. The small plate makes it look as if there is more food on the plate.
- Cut it in half. Serve half a sandwich instead of whole.
- Never order a super-size, mega-size or Extra anything. Get the regular or medium.

- Put chips and pretzels into single-serving size portions in zip bags instead of serving chips in a big bowl.
- Don't take your child to a buffet restaurant. It's just too easy to take too much.

Portions – what do they look like?

- A serving of meat (3 ounces) is the size of the palm of your hand <pictures, please>
- Fish serving of 3 ounces looks like a check book
- 1 cup of potatoes, rice or pasta looks like a tennis ball.

- 1 cup of vegetables is the size of a fist
- 1 ounce serving of cheese is about the size of your thumb
- 1 cup serving of milk, yogurt, or fresh greens is about the size of your fist
- 1 teaspoon of oil is about the size of your thumb tip

<it would be great to have a PDF for portion size, too! >

Summary:
There are many ways to help you and your children to make healthy eating choices. As a parent and a role model, you have a big part to play in your child's future. Use these tips to start today on a more healthy life.

"We must become the change we want to see."

Mahatma Gandhi

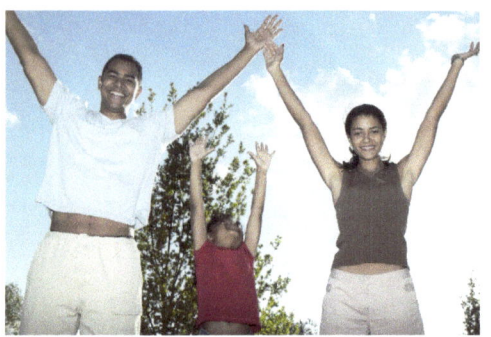

References

Anderson, RE, Crespo, CJ, Bartlett SJ, Cheskin, LJ, Pratt M. Relationship of physical activity and television watching with body weight and level of fatness among children: results from Third National Health and Nutrition Examination Survey. JAMA, 1998; 279 :938-942

J Am Diet Assoc. 2004; 104:660-677
Carlson, A., Lino M. Gerrior S., Basiotis, P. Report Card on the Diet Quality of Children Ages 2 to 9: Nutrition Insights, USDA Center for Policy and Promotion, 2001. September 2001

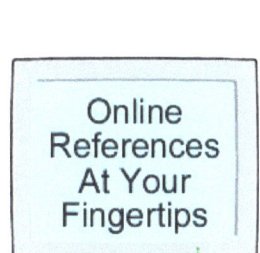

Resources

My Pyramid: Fun Internet page for kids ages 6 to 11 with a poster, coloring page, tracking page for kids, tips for families, eating and exercise tips, Blast Off Game where kids can reach Planet Power by fueling their rocket with food and physical activity., : http://www.mypyramid.gov/kids/index.html

Surgeon General information on overweight children

http://www.surgeongeneral.gov/topics/obesity/calltoaction/fact_adolescents.htm

Fast food calorie list:
http://www.thecaloriecounter.com/Foods/2100/Food.aspx

All about vegetables – tips for menus

http://www.fruitsandveggiesmatter.gov/benefits/index.html

Portion control and eating tips from the American Diabetes Association:
http://www.diabetes.org/for-parents-and-kids/diabetes-care/portion-control.jsp

Biography
Dr.Carleen Varga, RN, MSN, APN

Dr.Carleen Varga is an advanced practice nurse, with a masters of science in nursing and a doctorate in education She works at De Paul University in Chicago Illinois as a nursing professor and works as a consultant for the Illinois Nurses Association. Carleen served on Illinois Nurses Association and on the Continuing Education Advisory Board of the INA. She appeared on Channel 7 with her fitness studio and all her devoted members. Carleen has completed several studies relating to childhood obesity and has published both articles and books on exercise and fitness. Carleen Varga was a formal owner of Fitwize 4 Kids in Schaumburg, Illinois, a lifestyle center for children. Fitwize 4 Kids provided the opportunity for children to incorporate a healthy lifestyle for life. Carleen also volunteers at schools to teach health and nutrition to children. Carleen is married to John Varga, has two children, Katie and Michael. Carleen enjoys helping people, volunteering, and giving back to the community. Her mission is to educate and empower the children so they can become healthy and active adults for life.

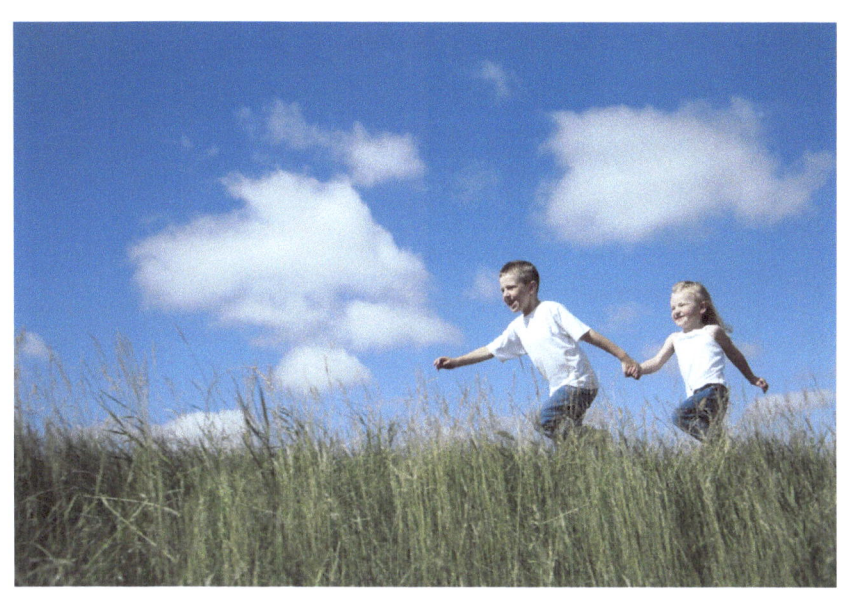

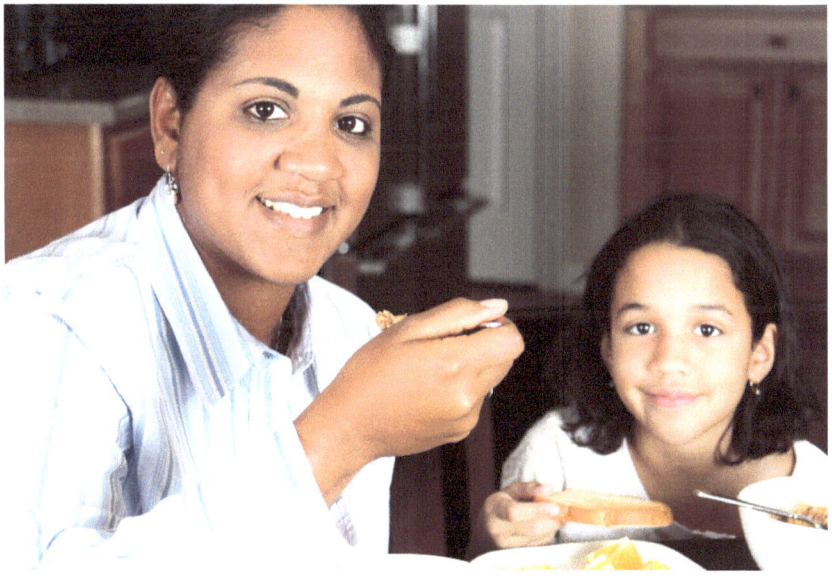

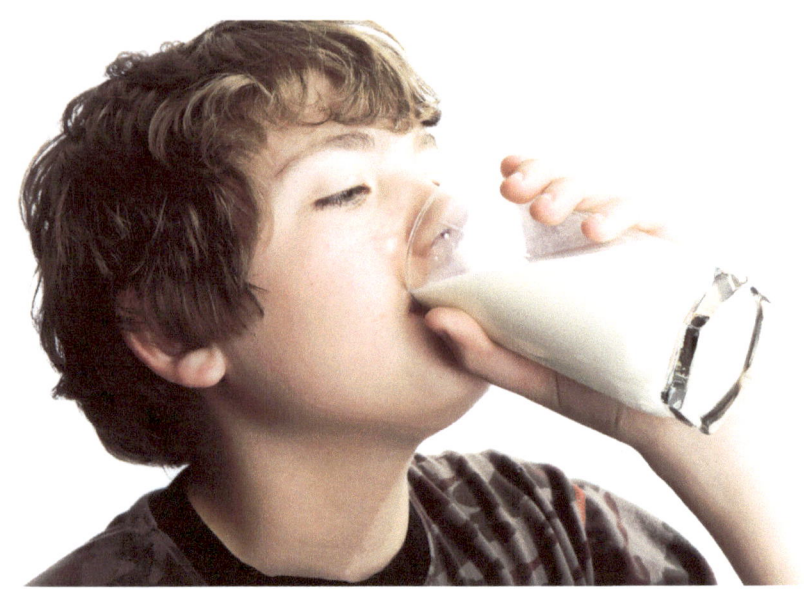

NO SODAS OR SUGARY DRINKS

Post Test

1. What can you do as a family to become more active?

a. Walking the dog
b. Playing Frisbee or flag football
c. Ice skating or rollerblading
d. All of the above

2. Which food is most healthy?

a. French Fries
b. Fresh fruit
c. Fruit Roll Ups
d. Ice Cream

3. What kind of things can you do as a parent to help your child eat well?

a. Eat dinner as a family
b. Go to a pizza place
c. Go to an ice cream parlor
d. Give cookies as a reward

4. Pick the healthiest choice for your child.

a. Apple Slices with peanut butter
b. Bag of chips
c. Plate of Nachos with cheese
d. Ice cream sundae

5. Which is the healthy choice?

a. Be active most of the days of the week
b. Eat white bread and white rice daily
c. Watch TV 3-4 hours per day
d. Eat high fat and sugar foods three times a day

6. What kind of bread is most healthy?
a. multigrain
b. wheat bread
c. 100% whole wheat flour
d. raisin

7. The healthiest way to eat a meal is:
   a. eating with your family
   b. eating in the car
   c. eating while you are reading

d. eating at a restaurant

8. Breakfast is not important
   a. True
   b. **False**

9. Low fat is always low calorie.
   a. True
   b. **False**

10. A portion size of meat is this size:
   a. A baseball
   b. **The palm of your hand**
   c. A grapefruit
   d. A DVD

Did you past the test ?   Good Job! Keep up the good work!

www.ingramcontent.com/pod-product-compliance
Lightning Source LLC
Chambersburg PA
CBHW050927290526
45792CB00002B/922